# DASH DIET RECIPES

*50 Heart Healthy*
**30 MINUTE**
*Low Fat*
*Low Sodium*
*Low Cholesterol*
*DASH Diet Recipes*
*to Help You Lose*
*Weight Fast and*
*Prevent Heart*
*Disease, Stroke,*
*Diabetes and Cancer*

**Gina Crawford**

**IMPORTANT**

The information in this book reflects the author's research, experiences and opinions and is not intended to replace medical advice.

Before beginning this or any nutritional or exercise regimen, consult your physician to be sure it is appropriate for you. Ask for a physical stress test.

# Table of Contents

# Introduction

The DASH diet is a lifelong well-balanced approach to healthy eating promoted by the National Institutes of Health that is based on nutrient-rich whole foods.

U.S News and World Report chose the DASH diet as the best overall diet, the healthiest diet and the best diet for diabetes for four years in a row.

The DASH diet reduces your sodium intake and increases your consumption of calcium, magnesium, potassium and fiber through a wide variety of whole foods that lower blood pressure.

Eating vegetables, fruits, whole grains, fish, lean meats, low-fat dairy and healthy fats is all part of the DASH diet healthy eating plan.

This book will help you achieve your DASH diet goals by providing delicious DASH diet 30 MINUTE recipes for breakfast, lunch and dinner plus snacks, appetizers, sauces, dips and dressings. It also includes nutritional information for each recipe!

*Enjoy!*

# Chapter 1

# What is the DASH diet?

*"Let food be thy medicine and medicine be thy food"*
*Hippocrates*

*Chapters 1 & 2 are taken from my*
*DASH Diet for Beginners book on Amazon*

The DASH diet is a well-balanced, lifelong approach to healthy eating that was discovered in research funded by the National Institutes of Health (NIH) to determine the role of dietary eating patterns on blood pressure.

Over the years a number of studies have proven that the DASH diet is not only effective for lowering blood pressure through diet but it is also effective in reducing the risk of cardiovascular disease, several types of cancers, stroke, heart disease, kidney stones, kidney disease, diabetes, heart failure and many other diseases. The DASH diet has also been shown to promote weight loss and improve overall health.

## The DASH diet is recommended by:

The Mayo Clinic

That American Heart Association

The American College of Cardiology

The Dietary Guidelines for Americans

US guidelines for the treatment of hypertension

The National Heart, Lung and Blood Institute (a part of the National Institutes of Health [NIH] of the US Department of Health & Human Services)

In January 2014 US News and World Report selected the DASH diet as the best overall diet, the healthiest diet and the best diet for diabetes for four years in a row.

The DASH diet was chosen by a distinguished panel of doctors for its healthy balance of food groups, its ability to improve health and its proven track record of successfully working time and time again.

# Chapter 2

# Characteristics of the DASH Diet

The DASH diet is not necessarily a "diet" rather it is a way of eating that promotes long term health. The USDA (U.S. Department of Agriculture) recommends the DASH diet as "an ideal eating plan for all Americans."

The NIH (National Institutes of Health) says that the DASH diet plan does more than promote good eating habits. It offers suggestions on healthy alternatives to junk food and processed food.

In addition to this, the creators of the DASH diet say that "not only is the DASH diet designed to bring down high blood pressure, it is also a well-balanced approach to eating that encourages people to lower their intake of sodium (salt) and increase their consumption of calcium, magnesium and potassium."

## The characteristics of the DASH diet include:

Lower sodium intake

Increased vitamins and minerals

Increased good fats

Increased fiber consumption

Reduction of alcohol and caffeine

Customizable sodium and caloric intake

## Lower sodium intake

The DASH diet provides guidelines for your sodium and caloric intake.

The standard DASH diet allows up to a maximum of 2300 mg of sodium per day and the low-sodium version of the DASH diet allows up to 1500 mg of sodium per day.

The average American diet contains up to 3500 mg of sodium per day.

## Increased vitamins and minerals

All your essential vitamins and minerals are provided on the DASH diet by the many fruits, vegetables, whole grains and other whole foods that you are encouraged to eat on the diet.

The diet also includes an ample supply of minerals like magnesium and potassium that help to lower or improve your blood pressure.

### Increased good fats

Consuming a lot of good fats and minimizing bad fats is highly encouraged on the DASH diet. Saturated and Trans fats should be replaced with lean meats, omega-3's from fish and seafood, low-fat dairy, nuts and seeds.

Good fats help to optimize our overall health by lowering bad cholesterol and increasing good cholesterol.

### Increased fiber consumption

The DASH diet recommends increasing your fiber consumption by eating several servings of fruits, vegetables and grains every day. This keeps you feeling full and helps to reduce blood pressure.

High fiber consumption also helps to maintain good blood sugar levels and it also encourages weight loss.

### Reduction of alcohol and caffeine

The DASH diet suggests limiting your intake of alcohol, soda, tea and coffee because they offer no nutritional value, typically contain a lot of sugar and they can elevate blood pressure.

## Customized sodium and caloric intake

In the same way that you can choose a 2300 mg/day or 1500 mg/day sodium intake DASH diet, you can also choose the most suitable caloric intake level for you. The DASH diet allows you to choose a diet of 1500 to 3100 calories per day.

The caloric intake that you choose will depend on your weight, activity level, whether you have high blood pressure now or want to prevent it etc.

If you are overweight you will likely opt for the lower caloric intake level. If you are active then you will likely choose the higher caloric intake level. If you have high blood pressure or at risk of developing high blood pressure due to family history etc. then you'll likely opt for the low sodium diet. Consider working with your doctor to come up with the best combination of sodium and calorie level for you.

# Chapter 3

# Breakfast

*"You don't have to cook fancy or complicated masterpieces – just good food from fresh ingredients."*

*Julia Child*

# Spiced Maple Syrup Hot Cakes

*Cinnamon is a good source of manganese. Those who take anti-seizure medications often test for low manganese levels. Osteoporosis and diabetes mellitus patients also have lower manganese levels than recommended.*

*Bananas protect the cardiovascular system, eyesight and build better bones. Be careful if you have an allergy to latex as the banana contains the same chitinase enzyme that causes latex allergies.*

*Serves 6*

## Ingredients

Maple syrup.....1/2 cup

Cinnamon.....1/2 stick

Whole cloves.....3

Pure old fashioned rolled oats.....1/2 cup

Water.....1 cup

Light brown sugar.....2 tablespoons firmly packed

Olive oil.....2 tablespoons

Whole wheat (whole-meal) flour.....1/2 cup

All purpose (plain) flour.....1/2 cup

Baking powder.....1 1/2 teaspoons

Baking soda.....1/4 teaspoon

Salt.....1/4 teaspoon

Ground cinnamon.....1/4 teaspoon

Fat-free plain yogurt.....1/2 cup

Banana.....1 peeled and mashed

Egg.....1 lightly beaten

## Directions

In a small saucepan combine the maple syrup, cloves and cinnamon stick. Place over medium heat and bring to a boil. Remove from heat and let steep for 15 minutes. Remove the cinnamon stick and cloves with a slotted spoon. Set the syrup aside and keep warm.

In a medium saucepan combine the oats and water over medium heat until the oats are tender and creamy. Stir in the olive oil and brown sugar then set it aside to allow the mixture to cool slightly.

Combine the whole-wheat flour, all-purpose flour, cinnamon, baking powder, baking soda and salt in a bowl. Thoroughly blend the ingredients together.

In a medium bowl whisk the milk, yogurt and banana together. Add this to the oats and stir until well blended. Beat the egg in. Add the flour mixture to the oat mixture and stir ingredients until moistened.

Place a nonstick frying pan or griddle over medium heat. When a drop of water sizzles on the pan it is ready to use.

Spoon a 1/4 cup of the pancake batter into the pan. Cook until the pancakes top surface bubbles and the edges turn light brown, about 2 minutes. Flip and cook until the bottom is nicely browned. Repeat with the remaining pancake batter.

Plate the pancakes. Drizzle with the warm maple, clove and cinnamon syrup. Serve.

## Nutritional analysis per serving

*Serving size: 3 pancakes*

Total carbohydrate 49 g

Dietary fiber 3 g

Sodium 243 mg

Saturated fat 1 g

Total fat 7 g

Cholesterol 32 mg

Protein 6 g

Monounsaturated fat 4 g

Calories 271

# Cranberry-Walnut Oatmeal

*Oatmeal is a whole grain that is rich in fiber. Eating more fiber reduces cholesterol and helps burn fat because it keeps you full longer.*

*Serves 4*

## Ingredients

Steel cut oats.....1 cup

Dried cranberries.....1/3 cup

Salt.....1/4 teaspoon

Ground cinnamon.....1/4 teaspoon

Water.....2 cups

Walnuts.....4 teaspoons chopped

Brown sugar.....4 teaspoons firmly packed

## Directions

In a saucepan, combine the steel cut oats, cranberries, salt, cinnamon and water. Bring to a boil over high heat then reduce the heat to low and simmer uncovered until the oats are tender and the mixture is creamy, about 20 minutes.

Spoon the oatmeal into four warmed bowls. Sprinkle each serving with 1 teaspoon of walnuts and 1 teaspoon of brown sugar. Serve immediately.

**Note:** Toasting walnuts brings out their nutty flavor. You can substitute the walnuts with raisins, apples, berries or any fruit you like.

### Nutritional analysis per serving

*Serving size: Approx 1 cup*

Total carbohydrate 39 g

Dietary fiber 5 g

Sodium 150 mg

Saturated fat 1 g

Total fat 4 g

Cholesterol 0 mg

Protein 5 g

Monounsaturated fat 1 g

Calories 212

# Raspberry Muffins

*Raspberries contain a phytonutrient called rheosmin also referred to as the raspberry ketone (pronounced key-tone). Studies have found that this enzyme accelerates weight loss.*

*Makes 12 muffins*

## Ingredients

Raspberries.....2/3 cup

Rolled oats.....1/2 cup

1 % low-fat milk.....1 cup

All-purpose flour.....3/4 cup

Grits.....1/4 cup

Wheat bran.....1/4 cup

Baking powder.....1 tablespoon

Salt.....1/4 teaspoon

Dark honey.....1/2 cup

Olive oil.....3 1/2 tablespoons

Lime zest.....2 teaspoons grated

Egg.....1 lightly beaten

## Directions

Preheat the oven to 400 °F (200 °C). Line a 12-cup muffin pan with wax paper or foil liners.

In a medium saucepan combine the oats and milk. Cook on medium heat and stir until the oats are tender and the mixture is creamy. Remove from heat and set aside while proceeding to the next step.

In a large bowl combine the flour, grits, bran, baking powder and salt.

In a small bowl whisk the eggs and set aside.

Add the honey, olive oil and lime zest to the oats mixture and mix all the ingredients together. Add the egg to the batter. Mix the batter until moistened but still slightly lumpy. Gently fold in the raspberries.

Use two tablespoons, one to scoop the batter and the other to push the batter into the muffin cups, filling each cup about 2/3 full.

Bake until the tops are golden brown, about 16 to 18 minutes. You should be able to insert a toothpick through the center and have it come out clean. If dough sticks to the toothpick, return the muffins to the oven for another minute or two.

Transfer the muffins to a wire rack and let them cool completely before serving.

**Nutritional analysis per serving**

*Serving size: 1 muffin*

Total carbohydrate 27 g

Dietary fiber 2 g

Sodium 126 mg

Saturated fat 0.5 g

Total fat 5 g

Trans fat <0.5

Cholesterol 16 mg

Protein 3 g

Monounsaturated fat 3 g

Calories 165

Sugars 11 g

# Buckwheat Pancakes with Strawberries

*Buckwheat is actually a fruit seed and not a cereal grain. It is related to the rhubarb and sorrel family which makes it a great substitute for people who have allergies to wheat or other grains.*

*Serves 6*

## Ingredients

Egg whites.....2

Olive oil.....1 tablespoon

Fat-free milk.....1/2 cup

All purpose flour.....1/2 cup

Buckwheat flour.....1/2 cup

Baking powder.....1 tablespoon

Sparkling water.....1/2 cup

Fresh strawberries.....3 cups sliced

## Directions

In a large bowl whisk together the egg whites, olive oil and milk.

In another bowl combine the all-purpose flour, buckwheat flour and baking powder and mix thoroughly.

Slowly add the dry ingredients to the egg white mixture as you alternately add the sparkling water. Make sure to mix between each addition until all the ingredients combine into a batter.

Place a nonstick frying pan or griddle over medium heat. Spoon 1/2 cup of the pancake batter into the pan. Cook until the top surface of the pancake bubbles and the edges turn lightly brown, about 2 minutes. Flip and cook until the bottom is nicely brown and cooked through, 1 to 2 minutes longer. Repeat with the remaining pancake batter.

Transfer the pancakes to individual plates. Top each with 1/2 cup sliced strawberries. Serve.

**Nutritional analysis per serving**

*Serving size: 1 pancake*

Total carbohydrate 24 g

Dietary fiber 3 g

Sodium 150 mg

Saturated fat - trace

Total fat 3 g

Cholesterol - trace

Protein 5 g

Monounsaturated fat 2 g

Calories 143

# Muesli Breakfast Bars

*Swiss physician and nutritional research pioneer Maximillian Bircher-Brenner introduced Muesli in the 1900s while preparing diets that were rich in fresh fruits and vegetables for his patients.*

*Muesli is a combination of rolled oats, fruits, and nuts. In Germany and Switzerland Muesli is considered a light evening dish.*

*Makes 24 bars*

## Ingredients

Pure old-fashioned rolled oats.....2 ½ cups

Soy flour.....1/2 cup

Fat-free dry milk.....1/2 cup

Toasted wheat germ.....1/2 cup

Sliced almonds or chopped pecans.....1/2 cup toasted

Dried apples.....1/2 cup chopped

Raisins.....1/2 cup

Dark honey.....1 cup

Natural unsalted peanut butter.....1/2 cup

Olive oil.....1 tablespoon

Vanilla extract.....2 teaspoons

Salt.....1/2 teaspoon

**Directions**

Preheat the oven to 325 °F (160 °C)

Lightly coat a 9 x 13-inch baking pan with olive oil.

In a large bowl combine the old-fashioned oats, dry milk, wheat germ, soy flour, almonds, apples, raisins and salt. Mix well with a large cooking spoon to blend and set aside.

In a small saucepan stir together the peanut butter, honey and olive oil over medium-low heat until well blended. Do not let the mixture come to a boil. Stir in the vanilla. Add the warm honey mixture to the dry ingredients and stir quickly until well combined. The mixture should be sticky but not wet.

Spread the mixture evenly into the prepared baking pan. Press firmly removing any air pockets.

Bake until the edges begin to brown, about 25 minutes. Let it cool in the pan on a wire rack for 10 minutes and then cut it into 24 bars.

When the bars are cool enough to handle remove them from the pan and place them on a rack to finish cooling. Store the bars in airtight containers then refrigerate.

## Nutritional analysis per serving

*Serving size: 1 bar*

Total carbohydrate 27 g

Dietary fiber 3 g

Sodium 75 mg

Saturated fat 1 g

Total fat 5 g

Trans fat 0 g

Cholesterol 1 mg

Protein 6 g

Monounsaturated fat 2 g

Calories 177

Sugars 11 g

# Cinnamon French Toast

*Cinnamon contains an organic compound called cinnamaldehyde that has an anti-clotting effect on blood flow. Cinnamaldehyde also has other traits including one used to prevent oral bacteria on the back of the tongue and throat. When administered in high doses it can aid in the treatment of melanoma cancers.*

*Serves 2*

## Ingredients

Egg whites.....4

Vanilla......1 teaspoon

Ground nutmeg.....1/8 teaspoon

Cinnamon bread......4 slices

Ground cinnamon.....1/4 teaspoon

Powdered sugar.....2 teaspoons

Maple syrup.....1/4 cup

## Directions

Preheat the frying pan or griddle over medium heat.

In a small bowl whisk the egg whites then add the vanilla and nutmeg. Whisk 2 minutes to make sure the ingredients are well mixed. Dip the cinnamon bread slices into the egg mixture. Turn to coat both sides.

Place the dipped bread on the frying pan or griddle. Sprinkle lightly with cinnamon. Cook until the bottom is golden brown and flip over. Repeat the cinnamon sprinkle and cook another 4-5 minutes or until the second side is toasty brown.

Place French toast on plates. Serve.

*Optional additions:* Add 1 teaspoon powdered sugar and 2 tablespoons maple syrup to each serving. Another great addition can include strawberries or even apple preserves.

## Nutritional analysis per serving

*Serving size: 2 slices French toast not including syrup, powdered sugars, or fruit additions*

Total fat 2 g

Calories 295

Protein 12 g

Cholesterol 1 mg

Total carbohydrate 56 g

Dietary fiber 1 g

Monounsaturated fat 1 g

Saturated fat < 1 g

Sodium 395 mg

# Buttermilk Waffles

*Does buttermilk contain butter? You would think that it does but it doesn't. It is actually the liquid that remains when the cultured butter making process is complete. Buttermilk in fact, is almost entirely fat-free. It is a great source of calcium, riboflavin, B12 and phosphorous.*

*Serves 6*

## Ingredients

Whole-wheat (whole-meal) flour.....1 cup

All-purpose flour.....1 cup

Baking powder.....1 teaspoon

Baking soda.....1/2 teaspoon

Sugar.....1 tablespoon

Buttermilk.....2 cups

Egg.....1

Egg whites.....4

Cooking spray

## Directions

Spray a waffle iron with cooking spray. Preheat the waffle iron while you prepare the batter.

In a large mixing bowl use a slotted spoon to combine the whole-wheat flour, all-purpose flour, baking powder, baking soda and sugar.

In a large bowl whisk together the buttermilk and one whole egg. Slowly add this to the flour mixture. Mix after each addition until fully combined.

In a large metal or glass bowl, use an electric mixer on high speed to beat the four egg whites until stiff peaks form. Gently fold the egg whites into the flour mixture.

Spoon or ladle about 3/4 cups of the batter into the waffle iron depending on the size of the iron. Spread slightly with a spoon and cook according to the manufacturer's instructions. Serve immediately.

**Note:** Try different toppings to change up the nutrients of this recipe. The waffles are great with fresh berries or cinnamon and peaches as opposed to syrup.

## Nutritional analysis per serving

*Serving size: 1 waffle*

Total fat 2 g

Calories 208

Protein 11 g

Cholesterol 39 mg

Total carbohydrate 37 g

Dietary fiber 3 g

Monounsaturated fat 1 g

Saturated fat 1 g

Sodium 281 mg

# Green Smoothie

*This smoothie is good any time of the day. I especially like it when I am on the go and want to get my nutrients from a drink rather than a full meal. It contains heart-healthy vitamins and delivers a powerful punch of antioxidants.*

*Serves 4*

## Ingredients

Banana.....1

Strawberries.....1/2 cup

Lemon....1 juiced, about 4 tablespoons

Blueberries or blackberries.....1/2 cup berries

Baby spinach .....2 cups

Fresh mint.....1 tablespoon or to taste

Ice water or ice.....1 cup

## Directions

Place all the ingredients in a blender and set to puree. If you like a crunchy cold mixture add ice cubes and set the blender to chop.

Pour into your favorite glass and enjoy!

## Nutritional analysis per serving

*Serving size: 6 ounces*

Total carbohydrate 12 g

Dietary fiber 2 g

Sodium 14 mg

Saturated fat - trace

Total fat - trace

Trans fat 0 g

Cholesterol 0 mg

Protein 1 g

Monounsaturated fat - trace

Calories 52

Sugars 0 g

# Chapter 4

# Lunch

*What you eat in private eventually is what you wear in public. Eat clean, look lean.*

# Rigatoni with Broccoli and Garlic

*By steaming the broccoli in this recipe you get broccoli's nutritional benefits for digestion while decreasing cholesterol. Broccoli also helps to detoxify your body while replenishing it with healthy vitamins.*

*Serves 2*

## Ingredients

Rigatoni noodles.....1/3 pound

Broccoli florets.....2 cups

Parmesan cheese.....2 tablespoons

Olive oil.....2 teaspoons

Garlic.....2 teaspoons minced

Freshly ground black pepper, to taste

## Directions

Fill a large pot 3/4 full with water and bring to a boil. Add the pasta and cook until al dente (tender yet a slight firmness remaining) 10 to 12 minutes. Drain the pasta.

While the pasta is cooking use a steamer and bring one inch of water to a boil. Add the broccoli to the basket, insert, cover and steam until tender, about 10 minutes. In a large bowl, combine the cooked pasta and broccoli. Toss with garlic, parmesan cheese and olive oil. Season with pepper. Serve immediately.

## Nutritional analysis per serving

*Serving size: Approx 2 cups*

Total carbohydrate 63 g

Dietary fiber 5 g

Sodium 111 mg

Saturated fat 2 g

Total fat 7 g

Trans fat 0 g

Cholesterol 4 mg

Protein 14 g

Monounsaturated fat 4 g

Calories 355

Sugars 0 g

# Sweet Herb-Crusted Cod

*If grilling is your thing, prepare the fish then place it in foil and seal. Grill for five minutes then flip and grill for another five minutes.*

*Serves 4*

## Ingredients

Herb-flavored stuffing.....3/4 cup

Cod fillets......4 - 4 ounces each

Honey.....1/4 cup

## Directions

Preheat the oven to 375 °F (190°C).

Lightly coat a 9x13 baking pan with cooking spray. Place stuffing in a freezer bag and seal closed. Crush with a rolling pin until it has a crumb texture.

Brush the fillets with honey and place in the bag of stuffing. Shake the bag gently to coat the cod evenly. Place the stuffing coated fillet on the baking dish and repeat with the remaining fillets.

Bake until the fish is opaque throughout, about 10 minutes. Serve immediately.

## Nutritional analysis per serving

*Serving size: 1 fillet*

Total fat 1 g

Calories 169

Protein 21 g

Cholesterol 49 mg

Total carbohydrate 18 g

Dietary fiber 1 g

Monounsaturated fat < 1 g

Saturated fat < 1 g

Sodium 162 mg

# Chinese Noodles with Spring Vegetables

*Reduced sodium soy sauce comes with a green lid and contains 25% less sodium than the regular brand. Less sodium means less salt.*

*Serves 4*

## Ingredients

Chinese noodles......1 package (8 ounces)

Fresh ginger.....1 tablespoon grated

Garlic cloves.....2 finely chopped

Reduced sodium soy sauce.....2 tablespoons

Oyster sauce.....2 tablespoons

Broccoli florets.....1 cup

Bean sprouts.....1 cup

Cherry tomatoes.....8 halved

Fresh spinach.....1 cup chopped

Scallions.....2 chopped

Crushed red chili flakes (optional)

Olive oil.....2 tablespoons

## Directions

Fill a large pot 3/4 full with water and bring to a boil. Add the Chinese noodles and cook until al dente, about 10 to 12 minutes. Drain the noodles. Set aside. Heat the olive oil in a large frying pan over medium heat. Add ginger and garlic and cook until slightly brown. Add the soy sauce, oyster sauce and broccoli and stir for about 3 minutes. Add the remaining vegetables and stir until they are warm. Plate the noodles and top with the stir-fried vegetables. Add red chili flakes.

## Nutritional analysis per serving

Total fat 9 g

Calories 270

Protein 9 g

Cholesterol 0 mg

Total carbohydrate 38 g

Dietary fiber 5 g

Monounsaturated fat 4 g

Saturated fat 2 g

Sodium 350 mg

# White Sea Bass with Dill Relish

*There are close to 475 different species of sea bass. The White Sea Bass is native to the west coast of the United States and its season runs from June to March.*

*Serves 4*

## Ingredients

White Sea Bass filets.....4 - 4 ounces each

White onion.....1 1/2 tablespoons chopped

Capers.....1 teaspoon drained

Fresh dill.....1 1/2 teaspoons chopped

Dijon mustard.....1 teaspoon

Lemon juice.....1 teaspoon

Lemon.....1 cut into quarters

## Directions

Preheat the oven to 375 °F (190 °C)

In a small bowl add the dill, capers, mustard, onion and lemon juice. Stir.

Place each fillet on a square of aluminum foil. Squeeze a lemon wedge over each fillet then spread 1/4 of the dill mixture over each piece of fish.

Wrap the aluminum foil around the fish and bake or grill until the fish is opaque throughout. Cook 10 to 12 minutes. Serve.

**Nutritional analysis per serving**

*Serving size: 1 fillet*

Total carbohydrate 3 g

Dietary fiber 1 g

Sodium 129 mg

Saturated fat < 0.5 g

Total fat 2 g

Cholesterol 46 mg

Protein 21 g

Monounsaturated fat < 0.5 g

Calories 119

# Chicken in White Wine and Mushroom Sauce

*Chicken is a great source of protein. For every 100 grams of chicken you get 30 grams of protein. In comparison, for every 100 grams of tuna, salmon and halibut there are 26 grams of protein.*

*This tasty dish is great when served over pasta. Add a side of freshly steamed vegetables for a nutrient rich, delicious meal.*

*Serves 4*

## Ingredients

Boneless skinless chicken breast.....4 - 4 ounces each

Olive oil.....2 tablespoons

Shallots.....4 thinly sliced

Fresh mushrooms.....1/4 pound thinly sliced

All-purpose (plain) flour.....1 tablespoon

White wine.....1/4 cup

Chicken stock.....1/2 cup low sodium

Fresh rosemary.....1 tablespoon (or 1 teaspoon dried rosemary)

Fresh parsley.....2 tablespoons chopped

**Directions**

Place the chicken breasts in a sealed Ziploc bag and pound with a mallet to flatten. Remove chicken and cut each piece in half lengthwise. Return to Ziploc bag and refrigerate until firm. When chicken is firm, get two frying pans ready to cook by placing one teaspoon of olive oil in each pan.

In a small bowl add the flour and wine then whisk until all the flour lumps are gone. Set aside.

Turn both of the frying pans to medium heat. In frying pan number one add the chicken breast. In frying pan number two, sauté the shallots for about 3 minutes. Return to frying pan number one and turn the chicken breast over. Go back to frying pan number two and add the mushrooms to the shallots. Stir while the two sauté together for another 2 minutes.

Get the bowl of mixed flour and wine. Whisk a few times and pour over the mushrooms and shallots. Add the chicken stock and stir. The chicken in the first pan should be a nice shade of brown on each side and cooked through with no pink remaining. Remove from heat and plate.

Go back to the mushroom and shallot pan and stir, making sure it has thickened nicely. Turn off the burner and spoon mixture over the chicken. Sprinkle with parsley and serve piping hot.

## Nutritional analysis per serving

*Serving size: 2 chicken breast halves*

Total fat 9 g

Calories 239

Protein 28 g

Cholesterol 66 mg

Total carbohydrate 6 g

Dietary fiber 0.5 g

Monounsaturated fat 5 g

Saturated fat 1 g

Sodium 98 mg

# Sun-Dried Tomato Basil Pizza

*Sun-dried tomatoes have high levels of antioxidants, lycopene and vitamin C. They are often used for tomato paste and tomato purees. The red plum tomato is used for sun-dried products.*

*Serves 4*

## Ingredients

12 inch prepared pizza crust purchased or made from mix.....1 crust

Garlic cloves.....4

Fat-free ricotta cheese.....1/2 cup

Dry packed sun-dried tomatoes.....1/2 cup chopped

Dried basil.....2 teaspoons

Thyme.....1 teaspoon

Red pepper flakes

Parmesan cheese

## Directions

Preheat the oven to 475 °F (250 °C).

Lightly coat a 12-inch round pizza pie baking pan with cooking spray.

Sun-dried tomatoes need to be reconstituted before using. Place them in a bowl and pour boiled water over them until they are covered in water. Let stand for 5 minutes or until soft and pliable. Drain and chop.

Place the pizza crust in a round pizza pie-baking pan. Arrange garlic, cheese and tomatoes on top of the pizza crust. Sprinkle basil and thyme evenly over the pizza.

Bake on the lowest rack of the oven until the pizza crust turns brown and the toppings are hot, about 20 minutes.

Cut the pizza into eight even slices and serve immediately.

Place the red-flaked pepper jar and the parmesan jar out for individual use.

## Nutritional analysis per serving

*Serving size: 2 slices*

Total fat 2 g

Calories 179

Protein 8 g

Cholesterol 8 mg

Total carbohydrate 32 g

Dietary fiber 2 g

Monounsaturated fat 0.5 g

Saturated fat - trace

Sodium 276 mg

# DASH Delicious Chicken Burritos

*This recipe calls for precooked chicken which means you won't have to wonder what to do with your leftover chicken anymore! Combining the precooked chicken with a vegetable dish offers a high amount of protein, vitamins A, C, E, K, B12, B5, B6, niacin, pantothenic acid, folate, choline, lycopene, and lutein zeaxanthin. The cheese assists with the digestion of the tomatoes wonder nutrient - lycopene.*

*Lycopene is the antioxidant compound that helps to reduce heart disease, macular degeneration and fat molecules that trigger heart disease. It is also beneficial in the prevention and treatment of some cancers.*

*Serves 4*

## Ingredients

*Sauce:*

Olive oil.....1 teaspoon

Red bell pepper.....1 chopped

Jalapeno pepper.....1 chopped

Celery.....2 chopped

Yellow onion.....1 chopped

Cumin seeds.....2 tablespoons

Grape tomatoes.....16 ounces

Fresh oregano.....2 tablespoons

Garlic cloves.....2 cloves chopped

*Burrito Filling:*

Chicken breast.....8 ounces precooked

Tortillas.....4 whole

Cheddar cheese (sharp)..... 1/2 cup shredded

Green cabbage.....2 cups shredded

## Directions

In a large skillet over medium-high heat add the oil and sauté peppers, celery, onion and cumin until lightly brown, about 10 to 15 minutes. Add tomatoes, oregano, and garlic. Continue to sauté until tomatoes blister and break open, about 5 to 10 minutes. Add contents to blender and puree until desired consistency.

Using the precooked chicken breast divide it among tortillas. Top with cheese, cabbage, and sauce. Roll up and enjoy.

**Note:** If you want the precooked chicken hot simply add it to the skillet in the last 5 minutes of the cooking time.

## Nutritional analysis per serving

*Serving size: 1 burrito*

Total carbohydrate 28 g

Dietary fiber 6 g

Sodium 276 mg

Saturated fat 4 g

Total fat 13 g

Trans fat 0 g

Cholesterol 63 mg

Protein 26 g

Monounsaturated fat 3 g

Calories 333

Sugars 0 g

# Spinach-Stuffed Sole

*Spinach and sole provide high levels of vitamin A, B2, B6, B12, E, K, manganese, folate, iron, copper, calcium and a slew of other vitamins and minerals.*

*Serves 2*

## Ingredients

Sole fillets.....2 - 5 ounces each

Olive oil.....1 teaspoon

Fresh spinach.....2 cups

Garlic.....2 teaspoons minced

Freshly ground black pepper.....to taste

Cooking spray

## Directions

Preheat the oven to 400 °F (200 °C).Lightly coat a baking dish with cooking spray.

Heat a skillet on medium heat. Add olive oil and warm. Add the garlic and sauté for one minute. Add the spinach and pepper then sauté until the spinach starts to wilt, about 2 minutes.

Spray the bottom of a glass-baking dish with nonstick spray. Place the fillets in the baking dish and spoon the spinach mixture into the middle of a fillet. Roll the fillet until it is seam side down. Repeat this with all the fillets.

Bake until the fish turns opaque throughout, about 8 to 10 minutes. Test the fish with a fork to see if it's ready. If the fish flakes it is ready to eat. If the fish doesn't flake, return it to the oven for a couple more minutes. Serve.

**Nutritional analysis per serving**

*Serving size: 1 fillet*

Total carbohydrate 1 g

Dietary fiber 1 g

Sodium 140 mg

Saturated fat 1 g

Total fat 5 g

Cholesterol 71 mg

Protein 27 g

Monounsaturated fat 2 g

Calories 157

# Chapter 5

# Dinner

*"This much I know. If you are what you eat*
*then I only wanna eat the good stuff."*
*Ratatouille*

# Roasted Salmon with Chives and Tarragon

*Salmon contains B3, B6, B12 selenium, protein, phosphorus, choline, pantothenic acid, biotin, and potassium. These nutrients are all essential for a healthy cardiovascular system, healthy joints, eye health and a decreased risk of cancer.*

*Serves 2*

## Ingredients

Organic salmon with skin.....2 - 5 ounce pieces

Extra virgin olive oil.....2 teaspoons

Chives.....1 tablespoon chopped

Fresh tarragon leaves.....1 teaspoon

Cooking spray

## Directions

Preheat the oven to 475 °F (250 °C).

Line a baking sheet with foil and light cooking spray.

Rub salmon all over with 2 teaspoons of extra virgin olive oil.

Roast skin side down about 12 minutes or until fish is thoroughly cooked.

Use a metal spatula to lift the salmon off the skin. Place salmon on serving plate. Discard skin. Sprinkle salmon with herbs and serve.

**Nutritional analysis per serving**

Total carbohydrate - trace

Dietary fiber - trace

Sodium 62 mg

Saturated fat 2 g

Total fat 14 g

Cholesterol 78 mg

Protein 28 g

Monounsaturated fat 7 g

Calories 241

# Lemony Seasoned Baked Cod

*Lemon is a great source of potassium, calcium, citric acid, magnesium, vitamin C and phosphorus. A great way to flush toxins out of your system is to start your day with a warm 8 ounce glass of lemon water. In order to do that simply juice half a lemon and add it to warm or room temperature water and drink. After you finish your lemon drink wait about 10-20 minutes before eating breakfast.*

*Serves 4*

## Ingredients

Cod fillets.....4 - 4 ounces each

Lemon.....1 cut into 4 wedges

Seafood-seasoning blend.....1 teaspoon

## Directions

Preheat the oven to 350 °F (175 °C).

Place foil on the bottom of a pan and spray lightly with nonstick cooking spray or if grilling divide foil into four sheets and spray each sheet with nonstick cooking spray.

Place cod fillets on the aluminum foil. Squeeze a lemon wedge over each fillet and sprinkle each with seafood-seasoning blend.

If grilling, wrap the aluminum foil pieces around the fish. Place in the oven or on the grill and cook until the fish is opaque throughout. Serve immediately.

## Nutritional analysis per serving

*Serving size: 1 fillet*

Total carbohydrate 3 g

Dietary fiber 1 g

Sodium 200 mg

Saturated fat - trace

Total fat 1 g

Cholesterol 49 mg

Protein 21 g

Monounsaturated fat - trace

Calories 105

# Pork Tenderloin with Herbes de Provence

*Herbes de Provence is a blend of spices that includes thyme, marjoram, rosemary, basil, fennel, sage and lavender. If you do not have this in your spice rack then it's definitely time to buy it. Try it with pork, chicken and vegetable platters. You're going to love it!*

*Serves 2*

## Ingredients

Pork tenderloin.....8 ounces trimmed of visible fat and cut crosswise into 6 pieces

Herbes de Provence.....1/2 teaspoon

Dry white wine.....1/4 cup

Freshly ground black pepper.....to taste

## Directions

Sprinkle the pork with black pepper and place it in a sealed freezer bag.

Thin the pork pieces by pounding them with a mallet or use a rolling pin until they are about 1/4-inch thick.

Heat a nonstick frying pan on medium-high heat. Add the pork chops to the pan. Sprinkle the pork chops with Herbes de Provence and cook for two to three minutes on each side until nicely brown. Place the pork on individual plates.

Pour the white wine into the hot frying pan. Cook and stir until boiling. Scrape the brown bits of cooked pork from the bottom of the pan. Pour the wine sauce over the pork and serve immediately.

**Nutritional analysis per serving**

Total fat 4 g

Calories 156

Protein 24 g

Cholesterol 74 mg

Total carbohydrate - trace

Dietary fiber 0 g

Monounsaturated fat 2 g

Saturated fat 1 g

Sodium 58 mg

# Balsamic Chicken Salad with Pineapple

*The chicken in this dish provides a great source of protein while the pineapple contains free radicals that fight colds, strengthen bones and improve gums. Pineapple also has anti-inflammatory properties as well as antioxidants for a healthy heart. The nutritional value of pineapple also includes immunity-boosting vitamin C as it prevents hypertension.*

*Serves 8*

## Ingredients

Boneless skinless chicken breast..... 4 - each about 5 ounces

Olive oil.....1 tablespoon

Unsweetened pineapple chunks.....1-8 ounce can drained except for 2 tablespoons of juice

Broccoli florets.....2 cups

Fresh baby spinach leaves.....4 cups

Red onions.....1/2 cup thinly sliced

*For vinaigrette:*

Olive oil.....1/4 cup

Balsamic vinegar.....2 tablespoons

Sugar.....2 teaspoons

Cinnamon.....1/4 teaspoon

## Directions

Heat the oil in a large nonstick frying pan on medium heat.

Cut each chicken breast into cubes.

Add the chicken to the heated olive oil and cook until golden brown, about 10 minutes.

In a large serving bowl combine the cooked chicken, sliced onions, pineapple chunks, broccoli and spinach.

*Vinaigrette:*

Whisk together the olive oil, vinegar and reserved pineapple juice. Add the sugar and cinnamon. Mix together then pour over the salad and gently toss to coat evenly. Serve immediately.

## Nutritional analysis per serving

Total carbohydrate 8 g

Dietary fiber 2 g

Sodium 75 mg

Saturated fat 1 g

Total fat 9 g

Cholesterol 41 mg

Protein 17 g

Monounsaturated fat 6 g

Calories 181

# Beef Stroganoff

*Lean cuts of beef like the round steak in this recipe contain important minerals like zinc, iron, selenium and phosphorus. This dish also works great served over brown rice or rice pilaf.*

*Serves 4*

## Ingredients

Olive oil.....1 tablespoon

Onion.....1/2 cup chopped

Boneless beef round steak.....1/2 pound cut 3/4 inches thick and all fat removed

Yolkless egg noodles.....4 cups uncooked

Fat-free.....1/2 can cream of mushroom soup (undiluted)

Water.....1/2 cup

All-purpose (plain) flour.....1 tablespoon

Paprika.....1/2 teaspoon

Fat-free sour cream.....1/2 cup

## Directions

Heat the oil in a nonstick frying pan on medium heat. Add beef and sauté for 3 minutes. Let the meat brown on all sides.

Add onions and sauté another 5 -10 minutes allowing the onions to turn translucent and the meat to get tender. Remove the mixture and set aside.

Fill a large pasta pot 3/4 full of water and bring to a boil. Add the noodles and cook until al dente, about 10 to 12 minutes. Drain the pasta.

Using the skillet with the steak and onion juices add the mushroom soup, water and flour then whisk together over medium heat. Stir until the sauce thickens, about 5 minutes.

Return the beef and onions to the frying pan with the sauce. Continue to cook over medium heat. Stir the mixture until warmed through. Remove from heat and add the sour cream. Stir.

To serve, divide the pasta among four bowls. Top with the creamy beef mixture and serve immediately.

## Nutritional analysis per serving

Total fat 6 g

Calories 302

Protein 24 g

Cholesterol 83 mg

Total carbohydrate 38 g

Dietary fiber 2 g

Monounsaturated fat 2 g

Saturated fat 2 g

Sodium 307 mg

# Halibut with Tomato, Basil and Oregano Salsa

*Halibut is a great source of magnesium. Magnesium is a natural calcium blocker which lessens the resistance of blood flow, oxygen flow and nutrients throughout the body.*

*Serves 4*

## Ingredients

Tomatoes.....2 diced

Fresh basil.....2 tablespoons chopped

Fresh oregano.....1 teaspoon chopped

Garlic.....1 tablespoon minced

Extra virgin olive oil.....2 teaspoons

Halibut filets......4 - 4 ounces each

Parmesan cheese.....optional

## Directions

Preheat the oven to 350 °F (150 °C). Lightly coat a 9 x 13-inch baking dish with cooking spray. In a mixer, combine the tomato, basil, oregano and garlic. Add the olive oil and chop another minute. Arrange the halibut fillets in the baking dish. Pour the tomato mixture over the fish. Place in oven and bake 10 to 15 minutes. Plate by pouring the tomato sauce over each fillet. Top with parmesan cheese.

## Nutritional analysis per serving

*Serving size: 1 fillet*

Total fat 5 g

Calories 160

Protein 24 g

Cholesterol 36 mg

Total carbohydrate 3 g

Dietary fiber 1 g

Monounsaturated fat 3 g

Saturated fat 1 g

Sodium 65 mg

# Pork Chops in Black Currant Jam Sauce

*Black currants grow on a five to six foot shrub that is native to Europe and Siberia. The black currant contains flavonoids that aid in the reduction and prevention of cancers and it also reduces inflammation. Black currents are an excellent source of vitamin A, B5, B6, B1, C, iron, copper, calcium, phosphorus, manganese, magnesium and potassium.*

*Serves 6*

## Ingredients

Black currant jam.....1/4 cup

Dijon mustard.....2 tablespoons

Olive oil.....2 teaspoons

Center cut pork loin chops.....6 - trimmed of all visible fat, 4 ounces each

White wine vinegar.....1/3 cup

Orange slices.....6

Mint leaves.....6

Freshly ground black pepper.....1/8 teaspoon

## Directions

In a small bowl, whisk together the jam and mustard.

In a large nonstick frying pan heat the olive oil over medium-high heat. Add the pork chops and brown on each side, about 5 minutes per side.

Top each pork chop with 1 tablespoon of the jam-mustard mixture spreading with the back of your spoon. Cover and cook for 2 additional minutes. Transfer the pork chops to the serving platter.

Cool the frying pan to a warm — not hot — temperature. Pour the white wine vinegar into the pan. Stir and remove the bits of pork and jam that seared to the pan. Stir the seared bits with the wine vinegar.

Pour the heated wine and vinegar sauce over each pork chop on the platter. Sprinkle with pepper and garnish with orange slices and mint leaves. Serve immediately.

**Nutritional analysis per serving**

Total fat 7 g

Calories 220

Protein 26 g

Cholesterol 71 mg

Total carbohydrate 12 g

Dietary fiber 1 g

Monounsaturated fat 4 g

Saturated fat 2 g

Sodium 198 mg

# Broiled Scallops with Sweet Lime Sauce

*Scallops are a great source of B12, magnesium and potassium. Magnesium helps the blood vessels to relax and let the blood flow easier. It also reduces blood pressure. Potassium works in the body to maintain blood flow. Scallops help to protect against stroke and fatal heart arrhythmias.*

*Serves 4*

## Ingredients

Bay or sea scallops.....1 pound rinsed and patted dry

Honey.....4 tablespoons

Lime juice.....2 tablespoons

Olive oil.....1 tablespoon

Lime peel.....2 teaspoons grated

Lime.....1 cut into four wedges

Cooking spray

## Directions

Position the broiler rack 4 inches from the heat source.

Preheat the broiler. Cover a broiler pan or cookie sheet with aluminum foil. Spray generously with cooking spray.

In a large bowl, whisk together the juice, honey and olive oil. Add scallops and turn gently to coat.

Arrange the sauce coated scallops in a single layer on the prepared broiler pan or baking sheet.

Broil for about 5 minutes. Turn the scallops over and broil for another minute to allow a golden searing.

Divide the scallops onto 4 plates. Spoon any juices from the broiler pan or baking sheet over the scallops.

Lightly sprinkle with grated lime peel and serve with a lime wedge.

## Nutritional analysis per serving

Total fat 7 g

Calories 220

Protein 19 g

Cholesterol 37 mg

Total carbohydrate 22 g

Dietary fiber 1 g

Monounsaturated fat 3 g

Saturated fat 1 g

Sodium 184 mg

# Chapter 6

# Salads

*Your skin replaces itself every 35 days. The liver, about a month. Your body makes these new cells from the food you eat. What you eat literally becomes YOU. You have a choice in what you're made of.*

*You are what you eat.*

# Simple Mango Salad

*Mangos help to fight against different types of cancers. They contain vitamin A, beta-carotene, alpha-carotene, beta-cryptoxanthin, potassium, vitamin B6, C, E and copper.*

*You can serve this salad over roasted chicken, chicken salad, oriental vegetables, tortellini salads or any salad that can use a little pizzazz!*

*Serves 6*

## Ingredients

Mangos.....3 pitted and cubed

Lime.....1 juiced

Red onion.....1 teaspoon minced

Jalapeno pepper.....1/2 seeded and minced

## Directions

Combine all the ingredients in a mixing bowl. Cover and place in the refrigerator for 10 minutes. Toss just before serving.

## Nutritional analysis per serving

Total carbohydrate 19 g

Dietary fiber 2 g

Sodium 10 mg

Saturated fat - trace

Total fat - trace

Cholesterol 0 mg

Protein 1 g

Monounsaturated fat - trace

Calories 75

# Asian-Style Vegetable Salad

*Bok Choy contains more beta-carotene and vitamin A than any other variety of cabbage.*

*Carrots are great at reducing the risk of cardiovascular disease. We typically associate carrots with the color "orange" but they actually come in fifteen different colors!*

*It is recommended that we eat richly colored vegetables. Red cabbage is a perfect example of a vegetable that has an intense, vibrant color. The red pigment intensifies the vegetables antioxidants and anti-inflammatory properties.*

*Serves 4*

## Ingredients

Carrot.....1/2 cup grated

Red bell pepper.....1/2 cup chopped

Bok Choy.....1 ½ cup chopped

Yellow onion.....1/2 cup sliced

Red cabbage.....1 cup sliced

Spinach.....1 ½ cups

Garlic.....1 tablespoon minced

Cilantro.....1 tablespoon chopped

Cashews.....1 ½ tablespoon chopped

Snow peas.....1 ½ cups

Low sodium soy sauce.....2 teaspoons

**Directions**

Rinse all the vegetables under cold running water then strain.

Cut the carrots, bell peppers, Bok Choy and yellow onion into thin strips.

To cut the cabbage and spinach put the knife across the grain and slice into narrow thin strips.

Mince the garlic. Cut the cilantro and cashews into slightly larger pieces.

Place cabbage, spinach, cilantro, cashews and snow peas in a large bowl. Drizzle with soy sauce. Toss well to combine. Serve.

## Nutritional analysis per serving

*Serving size: Approx 2 cups*

Total carbohydrate 14 g

Dietary fiber 4 g

Sodium 173 mg

Saturated fat 1 g

Total fat 4 g

Trans fat 0 g

Cholesterol 0 mg

Protein 3 g

Monounsaturated fat 2 g

# Two Bean Salad with Balsamic Vinaigrette

*Garbanzo beans or chickpeas contain molybdenum, manganese, folate, copper, fiber, phosphorus, protein, iron and zinc.*

*The highest nutrient content in the garbanzo bean comes from Molybdenum. Molybdenum ranks at 273.3 percent while zinc comes in at 22.8 percent. Molybdenum is common in legumes and a variety of other foods. The amount varies depending on the nutrient content of the soil it was grown in.*

*The high level of molybdenum in the garbanzo bean is well above the average daily recommendation of 45 micrograms for adults and 50 micrograms for pregnant women.*

*Serves 6*

## Ingredients

*For Vinaigrette:*

Balsamic vinegar.....2 tablespoons

Fresh parsley.....1/3 cup chopped

Garlic cloves.....4 - finely chopped

Extra virgin olive oil.....1/4 cup

Freshly ground black pepper.....to taste

*Mix in a bowl:*

Garbanzo beans.....1 can (15 ounces) rinsed and drained

Black beans.....1 can (15 ounces) rinsed and drained

Red onion.....1 medium

*Plating:*

Lettuce leaves.....6

Celery.....1/2 cup finely chopped

## Directions

To make the vinaigrette, use a small bowl and whisk together the balsamic vinegar, parsley, garlic and black pepper. Slowly add the olive oil while you whisk the ingredients. Set aside and allow the flavors to blend while you prepare the rest of the recipe.

In a large bowl combine the beans and onion. Pour the vinaigrette over the mixture and toss gently to coat. Cover and refrigerate to allow the flavors to marinate as the mixture cools.

To serve, put 1 lettuce leaf on each of 6 chilled plates. Divide the salad among the individual plates and garnish with chopped celery. Serve immediately.

**Nutritional analysis per serving**

*Serving size: Approx 1/2 cup*

Total carbohydrate 25 g

Dietary fiber 6 g

Sodium 170 mg

Saturated fat 1 g

Total fat 10 g

Trans fat 0 g

Cholesterol 0 mg

Protein 7 g

Monounsaturated fat 7 g

Calories 218

Sugars 0 g

# Triple Berry Spinach Salad

*Spinach contains phytonutrients like all other plants but it also contains over a dozen different flavonoid compounds.*

*There are three classes of flavonoids also known as bioflavonoids. The three classes are flavonoids, isoflavonoids and neoflavonoids. The classes represent the different molecular structures within the flavonoid family.*

*The flavonoids play a major role in reducing various cardiovascular diseases. They also have antibacterial properties.*

*Serves 4*

## Ingredients

Fresh spinach.....4 packed cups, torn

Fresh strawberries.....1 cup sliced

Fresh or frozen blueberries.....1 cup

Sweet onion.....1 small sliced

Pecans......1/4 cup chopped toasted

*Salad Dressing:*

White wine vinegar or cider vinegar.....2 tablespoons

Balsamic vinegar.....2 tablespoons

Honey.....2 tablespoons

Dijon mustard.....2 teaspoons

Curry powder.....1 teaspoon

Freshly ground black pepper.....1/8 teaspoon

## Directions

In a large salad bowl, toss together the spinach, strawberries, blueberries, onion and pecans.

In a small bowl combine the white wine vinegar or cider vinegar, balsamic vinegar, honey, Dijon mustard, curry powder and pepper. Whisk until well mixed.

Drizzle the dressing over the salad then toss to coat. Serve immediately.

## Nutritional analysis per serving

Total carbohydrate 25 g

Dietary fiber 4 g

Sodium 197 mg

Saturated fat 0.5 g

Total fat 5 g

Cholesterol 0 mg

Protein 4 g

Monounsaturated fat 3 g

Calories 158

# Spiral Pasta Salad with Pear and Soy Nuts

*Did you know that half the nutrients of a pear are in the skin? Pears can also reduce insulin resistance for people with Type 2 diabetes.*

*Water chestnuts are low in fat and high in complex carbohydrates. They provide dietary fiber and several essential minerals.*

*Soy nuts can help people with osteoporosis by increasing bone density. Soy nuts are also believed to help reduce cancer.*

*Serves 6*

## Ingredients

Whole-wheat spiral pasta.....4 ounces uncooked

Mixed greens.....6 cups

Fresh pears.....2 large cored and sliced

Golden raisins.....1/2 cup

Soy nuts.....3 tablespoons roasted, unsalted

Salt.....two pinches

*For the Dressing:*

Fresh or dried rosemary.....1 teaspoon

Ground cinnamon.....1/4 teaspoon

Salt.....1/4 teaspoon

Olive oil.....1/4 cup

## Directions

To make the dressing, add the rosemary, cinnamon, salt, balsamic vinegar and olive oil in a small glass dressing craft. Cover and shake thoroughly to blend. Place in refrigerator to chill and marinate while preparing the main ingredients.

Fill a large pot 3/4 full with water then add two pinches of salt. Add the pasta as the salt water comes to a boil. Cook until al dente 10 to 12 minutes. Drain the pasta and rinse under cold water.

In a large bowl combine the cooked pasta, mixed greens, pears, water chestnuts and raisins. Shake the dressing again and add it to the salad. Toss to coat. Divide the salad onto individual plates and top with soy nuts. Serve immediately.

**Nutritional analysis per serving**

Total carbohydrate 42 g

Dietary fiber 7 g

Sodium 122 mg

Saturated fat 1 g

Total fat 10 g

Cholesterol 0 mg

Protein 6 g

Monounsaturated fat 7 g

Calories 282

# Cherry Tomato, Basil and Pear Salad

*Five popular tomatoes are the Globe, Cherry, Heirloom, Roma, and Pear. The Globe tomato is a standard variant that is round and red. Cherry tomatoes belong to the cluster variant and have a juicy sweetness. Heirloom tomatoes ripen quickly and come in a large array of shapes and sizes.*

*Roma tomatoes or plum tomatoes are thicker skinned and have less seeds than other varieties. The Pear tomato comes from the cluster variant and tends to contain less juice than the Cherry tomato.*

*Serves 6*

## Ingredients

*For the Vinaigrette:*

Sherry vinegar or red wine vinegar.....2 tablespoons

Shallot.....1 tablespoon minced

Freshly ground black pepper.....1/8 teaspoon

Yellow pear tomatoes..... 1 1/2 cups halved

Red cherry tomatoes.....1 1/2 cups halved

Fresh basil leaves.....4 - cut into slender ribbons

Olive oil.....1 tablespoon

Salt.....1/4 teaspoon

## Directions

To make the vinaigrette, combine the vinegar and minced shallot in a mixing craft and let stand for 15 minutes. Add the olive oil, salt and pepper then cover and shake until well blended.

Toss all the tomatoes together in a large glass or stainless steel bowl. Do not use an aluminum or tin container since the acid in the vinegar can react to the metal producing an unwanted metallic flavor.

Pour the vinaigrette over the tomatoes, add the basil shreds and toss gently to coat. Serve immediately.

## Nutritional analysis per serving

Total fat 3 g

Calories 47

Protein 1 g

Cholesterol 0 mg

Total carbohydrate 6 g

Dietary fiber 1 g

Monounsaturated fat 2 g

Saturated fat 0 g

Sodium 108 mg

# Chapter 7

# Snacks

*"It is health that is real wealth and not pieces of gold and silver."*

*Mahatma Gandhi*

# Fruit Salsa 'n' Cinnamon Sweet Chips

*Give your tortillas a flavorful lift with some fruit and jam!*

*Serves 10*

## Ingredients

*For Tortilla Chips:*

Whole-wheat tortillas.....8

Sugar.....1 tablespoon

Cinnamon.....1/2 tablespoon

Cooking spray

*For Fruit Salsa:*

Fresh fruit such as apples, oranges, kiwi, strawberries, grapes or other fresh fruit.....3 cups diced

Sugar-free jam.....2 tablespoons any flavor

Orange juice.....2 tablespoons

## Directions

Preheat oven to 350 °F (175 °C).

Cut each tortilla into smaller single chip size wedges. Lay the pieces on a baking sheet. Make sure the chips are not overlapping. Lightly spray the tortilla pieces with cooking spray.

In a small bowl, combine sugar and cinnamon. Sprinkle the mixture of sugar and cinnamon evenly over the tortilla wedges. Bake for 10-12 minutes or until the tortilla pieces turn crisp. Place on a cooling rack while you prepare the salsa.

Mix the diced fruit together in a bowl.

In another bowl, whisk together the orange juice, honey and jam. Pour the sauce over the diced fruit and gently fold the sauce over the fruit.

Place a lid on the bowl or cover with plastic wrap and refrigerate for 15 minutes.

Serve as a dip or use as a topping over the cinnamon tortilla chips.

## Nutritional analysis per serving

*Serving size: Approx 8 chips and 1/3 cup salsa*

Total carbohydrate 21 g

Dietary fiber 3 g

Sodium 90 mg

Saturated fat - trace

Total fat 3 g

Trans fat 0

Cholesterol 0

Protein 2 g

Monounsaturated fat - trace

Calories 119

Sugars 3.5 g

# Cheesy Quesadillas

*I like to change this recipe up using whole-wheat tortillas one time and tomato tortillas the next. Tortillas are a great way to cut calories that a pizza crust or two slices of bread would raise. Quesadillas make a great snack, lunch or dinner.*

*Serves 16*

## Ingredients

Green chili peppers.....1 can (4 ounces) drained

Onion.....1/2 small, diced

Fat-free whole-wheat 10-inch tortillas.....8

Reduced fat Monterey Jack cheese.....2 cups (8 ounces)

## Directions

Preheat the oven to 350 °F (175 °C).

In a small bowl combine the drained green chili peppers with onion and cumin.

Sprinkle each tortilla with cheese. Divide pepper mixture among tortillas spreading it over the cheese. Top with another tortilla and place in a greased 9 x 13-inch baking pan.

Cover the pan with foil. Bake for 10 to 15 minutes or until the cheese melts.

Cut each tortilla into smaller pieces. Serve with your favorite salsa and sour cream.

**Nutritional analysis per serving**

*Serving size: 2 pieces*

Total carbohydrate 16 g

Dietary fiber 6 g

Sodium 200 mg

Saturated fat 1.5 g

Total fat 3 g

Cholesterol 10 mg

Protein 6 g

Monounsaturated fat 0.5 g

Calories 103

# Cranberry Spritzer

*Cranberry juice is a great source of vitamin C, E, K, copper and pantothenic acid. Cranberries also fight against tooth decay by reducing the amount of bacteria in the mouth.*

*Serves 10*

## Ingredients

Reduced calorie cranberry juice.....1 liter

Lemon juice.....1/2 cup

Carbonated water.....1 liter

Sugar.....1/4 cup

Raspberry sherbet.....1 cup

Lemon or lime wedges.....10

## Directions

In a large pitcher, mix together the lemon juice, cranberry juice, sugar and carbonated water. Refrigerate until cold.

Chill some glasses by rinsing them with water and putting them into the freezer wet. When the pitcher of juice is cold enough to serve, add the sherbet to the pitcher and stir.

Pour the spritzer into the chilled glasses and garnish with a lemon or lime wedge on the rim of the glass. Serve immediately.

**Nutritional analysis per serving**

*Serving size: Approx 1 cup*

Total fat 0 g

Calories 63

Protein trace

Cholesterol 0 mg

Total carbohydrate 15 g

Dietary fiber 0 g

Monounsaturated fat 0 g

Saturated fat 0 g

Sodium 21 mg

# Berry Creamy Parfait

*Strawberries help to prevent cardiovascular disease. They improve the regulation of blood sugars in Type 2 diabetes patients and they help to prevent certain kinds of cancers.*

*Blueberries help to lower cholesterol. They also cause cancer cells in the liver to self-destruct.*

*Serves 4*

## Ingredients

Fresh strawberries.....16 ounces, sliced

Fresh blueberries.....1 1/2 cups

*Creamy filling:*

Low-fat vanilla yogurt.....1 cup

Fat-free cream cheese.....1/4 cup

Honey.....1 teaspoon

Toasted Sunflower Seeds

## Directions

*Creamy Filling:* Beat the yogurt, cream cheese and honey in a bowl until fluffy.

*Assemble parfaits:* Place 1/3 cup strawberries in each parfait glass. Top with 3 tablespoons of creamy filling. Add 1/4 cup blueberries over the filling. Garnish with remaining fruit and sunflower seeds.

## Nutritional analysis per serving

*Serving size: 1 parfait glass*

Total carbohydrate 20 g

Dietary fiber 3 g

Sodium 116 mg

Saturated fat 0.4 g

Total fat 1 g

Cholesterol 2 mg

Protein 5 g

Monounsaturated fat 0.2 g

Calories 100

# Zesty Orange Soy

*Oranges contain vitamin B1, C, fiber, folate, potassium, copper, pantothenic acid and calcium. The white pulp in the orange that is closest to the skin is quite beneficial when it comes to lowering blood pressure and cholesterol. The orange also has antioxidants that fight disease, anti-carcinogens that fight cancers and compounds in the orange peel that lower cholesterol.*

*Serves 4*

## Ingredients

Orange juice.....1 1/2 cups chilled

Light vanilla soy milk.....1 cup chilled

Soft tofu.....1/3 cup

Dark honey.....1 tablespoon

Orange zest.....1 teaspoon grated

Vanilla extract.....1/2 teaspoon

Ice cubes......5

Orange slices.....4

## Directions

Rinse four tall serving glasses with water and place them in the freezer (wet) to chill. In a blender, combine the soymilk, orange juice, orange zest, tofu, honey, vanilla and ice cubes. Blend until frothy. Pour into chilled glasses. Garnish with an orange slice on the rim.

## Nutritional analysis per serving

*Serving size: Approx 1 cup (8 fluid ounces)*

Total carbohydrate 17 g

Dietary fiber 1 g

Sodium 21 mg

Saturated fat < 1 g

Total fat 1 g

Trans fat 0 g

Cholesterol 0 mg

Protein 3 g

Monounsaturated fat < 1 g

Calories 89

Sugars 4 g

# Chapter 8

# Appetizers

*If you don't recognize an ingredient, your body won't either.*

# Fruit Kebabs with Lemony Lime Dip

*Pineapples have numerous benefits. They prevent free radicals from forming, they have anti-inflammatory and anti-cancer benefits and they help to prevent atherosclerosis.*

*Strawberries are full of nutrients and can decrease the risk of developing Type-2 diabetes.*

*Kiwi has phytonutrients that protect DNA. Kiwi is also a good source of fiber as well as other nutrients.*

*Potassium is a well-known benefit of the banana.*

*Red grapes offer a whole list of heart-healthy nutrients that include lowering blood pressure and cholesterol levels.*

*Serves 2*

## Ingredients

Low-fat sugar-free lemon yogurt.....4 ounces

Lime.....1 for 1 teaspoon lime juice

Lime zest.....1 teaspoon

Pineapple chunks.....4 to 6

Kiwi.....1 peeled and diced

Banana.....1/2 cut into 1/2-inch chunks

Red grapes.....4 to 6

Wooden skewers.....4

## Directions

In a small bowl whisk together the lemon yogurt, lime juice and lime zest. Cover and refrigerate to allow the flavors to marinate as you prepare the rest of the recipe.

Thread one of each fruit onto a skewer. Repeat with the other skewers until the fruit is gone. Since Kiwi acts as a natural tenderizer place it next to the pineapple or grapes and avoid setting it right next to the banana to prevent premature browning.

Serve with the lemony lime dip.

To prevent fruit from browning, dip it in pineapple or orange juice.

## Nutritional analysis per serving

*Serving size: 2 fruit kebabs*

Total fat 1 g

Calories 160

Protein 4 g

Cholesterol 4 mg

Total carbohydrate 36 g

Dietary fiber 4 g

Monounsaturated fat - trace

Saturated fat < 1 g

Sodium 45 mg

# Apples with Peanutty Dip

*Apples are a great source of fiber and vitamin C. Eating an apple a day can help you maintain a healthy heart, reduce inflammation and lower cholesterol. Apple nutrients help to regulate blood sugar and they can also help prevent some kinds of cancer.*

*Serves 4*

## Ingredients

Fat-free cream cheese.....8 ounces

Orange juice.....1/2 cup

Brown sugar.....2 tablespoons

Vanilla.....1 1/2 teaspoons

Peanuts or walnuts.....2 tablespoons crushed

Apples.....4 medium or 8 small apples, cored and sliced

## Directions

Place the cream cheese on the counter and allow it to soften, about 5 minutes.

Crush the nuts and set aside. To make the dip, combine brown sugar, vanilla and softened cream cheese in a small bowl. Mix until smooth. Stir in the crushed nuts. Place sliced apples in another bowl. Drizzle orange juice over the apples to prevent browning. Serve the apples along with the dip.

**Nutritional analysis per serving**

*Serving size: 1/2 medium apple and 2 tablespoons of dip*

Total carbohydrate 18 g

Dietary fiber 2.5 g

Sodium 208 mg

Saturated fat 0.5 g

Trans fat 0 g

Total fat 2 g

Cholesterol 3 mg

Protein 5 g

Monounsaturated fat 0.5 g

Calories 110

Sugars 2 g

# Plum Tomato Crostini with Basil

*Tomatoes contain lycopene which is an antioxidant that is continually researched along with other nutrients to determine its effect on cancer cells. The tomato has one of the highest concentrations of lycopene though other fruits and vegetables also contain the antioxidant.*

*Serves 4*

## Ingredients

Italian bread.....1/4 loaf cut into 4 slices

Plum tomatoes.....4 chopped

Fresh basil.....1/4 cup minced

Olive Oil.....2 teaspoons

Garlic.....1 clove minced

Freshly ground pepper.....to taste

## Directions

Preheat the oven to 400 °F (200 °C).

Combine the chopped tomatoes, minced basil, olive oil, minced garlic and freshly ground pepper in a medium bowl. Cover and put in refrigerator for 20 minutes to allow the flavors to blend.

Take 4 slices of the Italian bread and place on a baking sheet. Toast in the oven.

Spoon the tomato mixture with any juices onto the toast. Serve at room temperature.

**Nutritional analysis per serving**

*Serving size: 1 slice*

Total carbohydrate 19 g

Dietary fiber 2 g

Sodium 172 mg

Saturated fat 0.5 g

Total fat 3.5 g

Cholesterol 0 mg

Protein 4 g

Monounsaturated fat 2 g

Calories 120

# Homemade Hummus

*Garbanzo beans are one of the best sources of insoluble fiber. Just 1/3 cup of garbanzos eaten daily has been proven to help regulate blood sugars and insulin levels.*

*Makes 3 cups*

## Ingredients

Garbanzo beans.....2 cans rinsed and drained except for 1/4 cup of liquid

Olive oil.....1 tablespoon

Lemon juice.....1/4 cup

Garlic cloves.....2 minced

Cracked black pepper.....1/4 teaspoon

Paprika.....1/4 teaspoon

Tahini (sesame paste).....3 tablespoons

Italian flat leaf parsley...2 tablespoons chopped

## Directions

In a blender or food processor, add the garbanzo beans and process to puree. Be sure to keep 1/4 cup of the canned garbanzo liquid set aside. Combine the olive oil, lemon juice, minced garlic, cracked black pepper, paprika, tahini and chopped parsley. Blend well.

Add the reserved liquid one tablespoon at a time until the mixture has the consistency of a thick spread. Serve immediately or cover and refrigerate until ready to serve.

Serve this Mediterranean spread with warmed whole-wheat pita bread or over Melba toast.

**Nutritional analysis per serving**

*Serving size: 2 tablespoons*

Total fat 2 g

Calories 48

Protein 2 g

Cholesterol 0 mg

Total carbohydrate 6 g

Dietary fiber 2 g

Monounsaturated fat 1 g

Saturated fat < 1 g

Sodium 106 mg

# Chipotle Spiced Shrimp

*Shrimp contains astaxanthin which gives shrimp its pinkish color. This carotenoid offers anti-inflammatory and antioxidant benefits that can suppress inflammation-messaging molecules like the ones in tumor necrosis and interleukin B1. This can reduce colon cancer and help the immune related problems of diabetes.*

*Serves 4*

## Ingredients

Shrimp (uncooked).....1/2 pound peeled and deveined (about 32 shrimp)

Tomato paste.....2 tablespoons

Water.....1/2 teaspoon

Olive oil.....1/2 teaspoon

Garlic.....1/2 teaspoon minced

Chipotle chili powder.....1/2 teaspoon

Fresh oregano.....1/2 teaspoon chopped

## Directions

Rinse shrimp in a strainer then pat them dry with a paper towel. Set aside on a plate.

To make the marinade, whisk together the tomato paste, water and oil in a small bowl. Add garlic, chili powder and oregano. Mix well.

Using a brush, spread the marinade (it will be thick) on both sides of the shrimp. Place in the refrigerator.

Prepare a hot fire in a charcoal grill or heat a gas grill or broiler (grill). Away from the heat source, lightly coat the grilling rack or broiler pan with cooking spray. Position the grilling rack 4 to 6 inches from the heat source.

Put the shrimp in a grill basket, foil coated with cooking spray or on skewers and place on the grill. Turn the shrimp after 3 to 4 minutes. The cooking time varies depending on the heat of the fire so watch carefully.

Transfer to a plate and serve immediately.

## Nutritional analysis per serving

*Serving size: 8 shrimp*

Total fat 2 g

Calories 73

Protein 12 g

Cholesterol 85 mg

Total carbohydrate 3 g

Dietary fiber 1 g

Monounsaturated fat 1 g

Saturated fat - trace

Sodium 151 mg

# Tomato Basil Bruschetta

*Tomatoes are a terrific choice if you are trying to lose weight. They are also beneficial in cancer prevention. One interesting thing about the tomato is that the more you cook it the higher the nutrient value climbs. Most fruits and vegetables lose their full level of nutritional value when cooked for longer periods but not the tomato!*

*Serves 6*

## Ingredients

Whole grain baguette.....1/2 cut into six 1/2 inch thick diagonal slices

Fresh basil......2 tablespoons chopped

Fresh parsley.....1 tablespoon chopped

Garlic cloves.....2 minced

Tomatoes.....3 diced

Fennel.....1/2 cup diced

Olive oil.....1 teaspoon

Balsamic vinegar.....2 teaspoons

Freshly ground black pepper.....1 teaspoon

Parmesan cheese......3 tablespoons

**Directions**

Dice the tomatoes and place them in a medium bowl. Add chopped basil, parsley, minced garlic, diced fennel, olive oil, balsamic vinegar and black pepper. Stir. Place in the refrigerator for 20 minutes to let the flavors blend.

Preheat the oven to 400 °F (200 °C).

Take the whole grain baguette and cut it into thick diagonal slices about 1/2 inch thick. Set on a baking sheet and put it into the oven. Toast the baguettes until they are lightly browned. Sprinkle with parmesan cheese while hot out of the oven. Transfer to a salsa serving platter.

Add the tomato basil mixture to the platter in a serving bowl with a spoon. Serve immediately.

## Nutritional analysis per serving

*Serving size: 1 slice*

Total carbohydrate 20 g

Dietary fiber 4 g

Sodium 123 mg

Saturated fat < 0.5 g

Total fat 2 g

Trans fat 0 g

Cholesterol 0 mg

Protein 3 g

Monounsaturated fat 1 g

Calories 110

Sugars 0 g

# Chapter 9

# Sauces, Dressings, and Dips

*"The food you eat can either be the safest and most powerful form of medicine or the slowest form of poison."*

*Ann Wigmore*

# Raspberry Coulis

*Raspberries are a great source of vitamin C, E, K, manganese, fiber, copper, pantothenic acid, biotin, magnesium, folate, omega-3 and potassium. Raspberries also raise metabolism levels to combat obesity.*

*Organic raspberries contain higher levels of antioxidants that help prevent cancer. They also have anti-inflammatory agents and phytonutrients.*

*Raspberry Coulis is terrific served over your favorite fruits, swirled into yogurt or drizzled over a sponge or pound cake.*

*Makes about 1 cup*

## Ingredients

Fresh raspberries.....3 cups

Honey.....2 tablespoons

Balsamic vinegar.....1 tablespoon

Ground cinnamon.....1/4 teaspoon

Ground nutmeg.....generous pinch

## Directions

If you do not have a food processor use a blender to combine all the ingredients. Once blended, turn the blender to puree until the ingredients yield a smooth mixture. Get it as smooth as you can before passing it through the meshed strainer.

Pass the purée through a fine-mesh strainer into a bowl. Press firmly on the mixture with a rubber spatula, wooden spoon or press with a small 1/4 cup measuring device against the sides to extract all the juice.

Scrape the inside of the strainer periodically to dislodge any seeds that may be plugging the holes. Keep pushing the pulp firmly through the strainer until all that is left is a small number of seeds. Cover the purée and refrigerate until ready to use.

## Nutritional analysis per serving

*Serving size: 1/4 cup*

Total carbohydrate 21 g

Dietary fiber 6 g

Sodium 2 mg

Saturated fat - trace

Total fat 0.5 g

Trans fat 0

Cholesterol 0 mg

Protein 1 g

Monounsaturated fat - trace

Calories 85

Sugars 9 g

# Artichoke Dip

*Artichokes are great for calming the stomach or relieving stomach pains. Research has also found that artichokes can help reduce high cholesterol. If you have gallstones check with your doctor before eating artichokes. If you have allergies to ragweed, chrysanthemums, marigolds or daises you should check with your doctor as well since artichokes come from the same family of flowers.*

*Serves 8*

## Ingredients

Artichoke hearts.....2 cups

Spinach.....4 cups chopped

Thyme.....1 teaspoon minced

Garlic.....2 cloves minced

Fresh parsley.....1 tablespoon minced

White beans.....1 cup prepared

Parmesan cheese.....2 tablespoons

Low-fat sour cream.....1/2 cup

Freshly ground black pepper.....1 tablespoon

## Directions

Preheat the oven to 350 °F (175 °C) Mix the ingredients together in a large bowl. Transfer to a glass or ceramic dish and bake for 20 minutes. Serve warm with whole-grain bread, crackers or vegetables for dipping.

## Nutritional analysis per serving

*Serving size: Approx 1/2 cup*

Total carbohydrate 14 g

Dietary fiber 6 g

Sodium 71 mg

Saturated fat 1 g

Total fat 2 g

Trans fat 0 g

Cholesterol 6 mg

Protein 5 g

Monounsaturated fat 1 g

Calories 94

Sugars 0 g

# Avocado Dip

*Avocados help to lower bad cholesterol and increase good cholesterol. They are also a good source of dietary fiber, vitamin B6, C, E, and K.*

*Serves 4*

## Ingredients

Fat-free sour cream.....1/2 cup

Onion.....2 teaspoons chopped

Hot sauce.....1/8 teaspoon

Avocado.....1 peeled, pitted and mashed

## Directions

Add the avocado to a medium bowl. Use a mixer on low to medium speed and mash the avocado. If you prefer a lumpier dip, use a hand-held masher or large spoon.

Add the chopped onion, hot sauce and the fat-free sour cream and combine. Serve.

## Nutritional analysis per serving

*Serving size: 1/4 cup*

Total carbohydrate 8 g

Dietary fiber 2 g

Sodium 51 mg

Saturated fat 1 g

Total fat 5 g

Trans fat 0 g

Cholesterol 3 mg

Protein 2 g

Monounsaturated fat 3 g

Calories 85

Sugars 0 g

# Guacamole

*Avocados contain an antioxidant named Lutein. Lutein helps prevent eye diseases such as cataracts and macular degeneration.*

*Serves 8*

## Ingredients

Avocado.....1 diced, about 1/2 cup

Beans (black or pinto).....1/2 can drained and rinsed

Ground cumin.....2 teaspoons

Lime.....1 juiced, about 2 tablespoons

Cayenne, chipotle or ancho chili powder.....1/4 teaspoon

Tomato.....1 large diced

Shallot.....1 minced

## Directions

In a medium bowl, add the avocado, beans, cumin, juice and cayenne pepper. Use a hand-held mixer on low speed and mix, about 2 minutes.

Add the tomato and shallots then mix with a spoon to combine. Serve.

**Nutritional analysis per serving**

*Serving size: Approx 1/4 cup (4 tablespoons)*

Total carbohydrate 6 g

Dietary fiber 2 g

Sodium 4 mg

Saturated fat 0.5 g

Total fat 3 g

Trans fat 0 g

# Delicious Glaze for Chicken, Fish or Vegetables

*Lemons and limes are great sources of vitamin C and folate. Vitamin C neutralizes free radicals while folate works at the cellular level. Folate is also helpful in correcting anemia.*

*Serves 4*

### Ingredients

Lemon or lime.....1 teaspoon, juiced

Lemon or lime zest.....1 teaspoon grated

Chicken broth.....1/2 cup unsalted

Fresh parsley.....1 tablespoon chopped

Sugar.....1 tablespoon

Cornstarch.....2 teaspoons

### Directions

In a microwavable bowl, combine juice, zest, broth and sugar. Pour half the mixture back into the broth cup and add the cornstarch.

Stir the cornstarch mixture making sure there are no lumps. Pour back into the microwavable bowl and whisk.

Add the parsley and whisk until mixed.

Microwave on high until clear and thick, about 1 to 2 minutes. Stir before serving.

**Nutritional analysis per serving**

*Serving size: 2 tablespoons*

Total fat 0 g

Calories 24

Protein 1 g

Cholesterol 0 mg

Total carbohydrate 5 g

Dietary fiber - trace

Monounsaturated fat 0 g

Saturated fat 0 g

Sodium 20 mg

# Cranberry Orange Glaze

*Cranberries contain fiber, manganese, vitamins C, E, K, copper and pantothenic acid. Most people know about the cranberries ability to protect against urinary tract infection but many do not realize that cranberries also act as an anti-inflammatory that benefits the cardiovascular system.*

*Serves 4*

## Ingredients

Fresh cranberries.....1 cup chopped

Unsweetened orange juice.....2/3 cup divided

Cornstarch.....1 tablespoon

Sugar substitute.....to taste

## Directions

In a small cup, add one-tablespoon cornstarch and 1/3 cup of orange juice. Stir until cornstarch dissolves. Set aside.

In a small saucepan, combine the cranberries and 1/3 cup unsweetened orange juice. Heat on medium until slow rolling bubbles form then add the orange juice and cornstarch mixture to the pan. Stir the mixture as you allow the sauce to heat back up to rolling bubbles. You should notice a change in the mixtures thickness as it forms the glaze. Remove from the heat and let it cool while you plate the main course.

Add the sugar substitute to the cooled glaze. The sugar substitute should be equivalent to one teaspoon of sugar. The glaze will be tart. Serve over chicken, turkey or pork. This glaze can also be used for grilling, roasting or as a marinade.

**Nutritional analysis per serving**

Total fat 0 g

Calories 38

Protein 0 g

Cholesterol 0 mg

Total carbohydrate 9 g

Dietary fiber 1g

Monounsaturated fat 0 g

Saturated fat 0 g

Sodium 1 mg

# Peach Honey Spread

*Peaches are full of vitamins, minerals, protein and beta-carotene that help prevent cancer. The fiber content of peaches assists with healthy digestion. The peach alkaline levels aid in the relief of digestive abnormalities and peaches also contain properties that bring down cholesterol levels.*

*This tasty spread is great with pancakes, waffles, roasted pork, roasted chicken and even on toast!*

*Serves 6*

## Ingredients

Fresh cranberries.....1 cup chopped

Unsweetened peach halves.....1 – 15 ounce can, drained

Honey.....2 tablespoons

Cinnamon.....1/2 teaspoon

## Directions

Put the drained unsweetened peach halves in a mixer and set it to chop. When the peaches have a chunky texture comparable to applesauce, transfer them to a large bowl. Add the honey and cinnamon to the peaches. Mix with a large spoon.

Chill in the refrigerator until ready to serve or serve warm over your favorite dish.

**Nutritional analysis per serving**

*Serving size: 1/3 cup*

Total fat 0 g

Calories 60

Protein 0.5 g

Cholesterol 0 mg

Total carbohydrate 16 g

Dietary fiber 1 g

Monounsaturated fat 0 g

Saturated fat 0 g

Sodium 4 mg

# Mango Salsa

*Ripe mangos are a delicious heart-healthy food. Mangos contain folate, niacin, pantothenic acid, riboflavin, thiamin, vitamins A, B6, C, E, K, potassium, calcium, copper, iron, magnesium, manganese, zinc and phytonutrients.*

*Serves 4*

## Ingredients

Mangos.....2 cubed

Red onion.....1/2 small minced, about 1/3 cup

Cilantro.....2 tablespoons minced

Red Fresno peppers.......3 minced, about 1/3 cup

Lime zest and juice.....1 lime

Olive oil.....1 tablespoon

## Directions

Take your mango and put it stem side down on the cutting board. Slice in three lengthwise sections leaving the flat yet oblong pit to the center section. Take the outer sections and cut cross sections down to the mango skin. The mango should scrape right off the skin into a large bowl. Repeat this step for both mangos.

Add minced red onion, cilantro, Fresno peppers, olive oil, lime zest and juice to the bowl. Mix thoroughly with the mango and serve over grilled chicken, tortillas or with black beans.

**Nutritional analysis per serving**

*Serving size: Approx 2/3 cup*

Total carbohydrate 15 g

Dietary fiber 2 g

Sodium 2 mg

Saturated fat 0.5 g

Total fat 4 g

Trans fat 0 g

Cholesterol 0 mg

Protein 1 g

Monounsaturated fat 2.5 g

Calories 100

Sugars 0 g

# Mushroom Sauce with Chives and Sherry

*Button mushrooms contain niacin, riboflavin, folate, phosphorus, iron, pantothenic acid, zinc, potassium, copper, magnesium, B6, selenium and thiamin.*

*A serving of button mushrooms has more potassium than a banana. The nutrients in the button mushroom help protect the cardiovascular system and reduce blood pressure.*

*Tantalize your taste buds with this flavorful mushroom sauce served over roasted chicken, baked pork chops, a lean strip of steak, vegetables or rice.*

*Serves 10*

## Ingredients

Fat-free milk.....2 cups

Olive oil.....2 teaspoons

Onion.....1 small, diced

Fresh mushrooms.....1 ½ cups sliced

All-purpose (plain) flour.....2 tablespoons

Chives.....1 tablespoon chopped

Sherry.....1 teaspoon

Freshly ground black pepper.....to taste

**Directions**

Slowly warm the milk in a small saucepan.

Add the olive oil to a nonstick skillet over medium heat. Drop an onion into the oil. It should sizzle lightly around the edges. Adjust the heat to sauté if needed and add the remaining onions cooking about 2-3 minutes until they are tender.

Add the sliced mushrooms and sauté another 3 minutes. Stir in the flour and continue to cook another 2-3 minutes.

Whisk in the warmed milk as you continue to cook. Make sure the flour has mixed evenly so there are no lumps.

Stir frequently until thickened, about 3 minutes.

Add chives, pepper and sherry. Mix. Reduce heat to simmer if you want to keep warm until serving. Stir periodically to make sure that nothing sticks to the bottom.

**Nutritional analysis per serving**

*Serving size: 1/4 cup*

Total fat 1 g

Calories 41

Protein 2 g

Cholesterol 1 mg

Total carbohydrate 6 g

Dietary fiber 0 g

Monounsaturated fat 1 g

Saturated fat - trace

Sodium 25 mg

# Other books by Gina Crawford

DASH Diet for Beginners

The 5:2 Diet for Beginners

5:2 Diet 30 Minute Recipes

Mediterranean Diet for Beginners

Mediterranean Diet Cookbook

Sugar Detox for Beginners

Sugar Free Recipes

Paleo for Beginners

## *Available on Amazon*

# Conclusion

I love all the recipes in this book and I know from experience that if you stick with the DASH diet and eat the foods suggested in this book you will lose weight and improve your health.

For more information on the DASH diet please search "DASH diet for Beginners - Gina Crawford" on Amazon under "Books" or "Kindle books." My best-selling "DASH diet for Beginners Quick Start Guide" will give you all the information you need to make this diet work for you!

Here's to a lifetime of great health and vitality!

# About Gina Crawford

Understanding what it takes to live a healthy lifestyle, eat right, achieve your goal weight and love your life shouldn't be complicated. Your time is valuable and the last thing you need is to tackle a 300 page book on how to get your health, weight and life on track. If you're like most people, you just want the facts in bite-sized, easy to understand pieces that you can apply to your life TODAY!

My name is Gina Crawford. I am a health and "all things natural" enthusiast, author, mother and wife. Years ago I was overweight, exhausted, unhappy and desperately aching for a better life. One day, gruelingly tired of my situation, I started researching everything I could on health and transforming my life. Often I felt overwhelmed by the amount of information and the changes I had to make, but I persevered and managed to turn my life around one book and one bite at a time.

Now I'm determined to share what I've learned in an easy, non-overwhelming, "no fluff, no filler, straight to the point" kind of way that will allow others to achieve maximum results in a short amount of time.

I am passionate about every book I write and my goal with each book is to make it simple and concise yet power-packed with the necessary information you need to transform your life. I have learned first-hand the incredible value of healing ourselves with natural organic foods, natural remedies, exercise and a positive mindset.

When I'm not writing, I love spending time with my family, cooking, walking, biking and reading.

My hope is that my books will help you live a healthier, better, more passionate, alive life!

Happy reading!

48665153R00085

Made in the USA
Lexington, KY
09 January 2016